*The Ancient Egyptian
Medicine Plant*

ALOE VERA
HANDBOOK

Max B. Skousen

Healthy Living Publications
Summertown, Tennessee

© 1992 Max B. Skousen

Cover photo and design: Warren Jefferson

Published in the United States by
Healthy Living Publications
an imprint of Book Publishing Company
P.O. Box 99
Summertown, TN 38483
1-888-260-8458
www.bookpubco.com

ISBN10 1-57067-169-9
ISBN13 978-1-57067-169-2

Printed in the United States

15 14 13 12   9 8 7 6

The Aloe Vera Handbook is intended solely for informational and educational purposes and not as medical counseling. Please consult a medical or health professional if you have questions about any conditions related to your health. The publisher and author are not responsible for any adverse effects or consequences resulting from the use of any of the suggestions or preparations discussed in this book.

Book Publishing Co. is a member of Green Press Initiative. We chose to print this title on paper with 100% postconsumer recycled content and processed chlorine free, which prevented the waste of the following natural resources:

BOOK PUBLISHING COMPANY

5 trees
146 lbs of solid waste
2,411 gallons of water
501 lbs of greenhouse gases
2 million BTU

green press INITIATIVE

For more information visit: <www.greenpressinitiative.org> Savings calculations from the Environmental Defense Paper Calculator at <www.edf.org/papercalculator>

ALOE VERA HANDBOOK

At a party attended by the noted writer Gertrude B. Foster, a guest thoughtlessly folded back the cover of a pack of paper matches to strike a light. The flare ignited the whole packet and before he could drop it in an ash tray his thumb and forefinger were painfully burned. The hostess quickly seized a cactus-like plant from the window sill, cut off a succulent leaf, and applied the cut end to the burn. A transparent mucilaginous gel from the leaf brought instant relief of the pain and dried in a few minutes without stickiness.

As other guests gathered around to watch this unusual first aid treatment, the hostess explained, "I always keep Aloe in the house for first aid. I remember how my mother in Sweden used it in the kitchen for burns."

The next day, Mrs. Foster called the guest who had been burned and treated with a house plant to see how he was. He reported that the skin was not in the least red and the pain had gone completely. After such a vivid demonstration of its worth, he wanted to know more about the amazing plant.

The succulent leaves of Aloe Vera are one of nature's perfect packaging miracles. Break a leaf off the fleshy stem from which a fan of sessile leaves radiate, and the plant quickly seals in the vital juices. Even the cut segment will heal over the end where it is sliced and retain its plumpness to remain green for several days. In a refrigerator it keeps for two or three weeks. The transparent pulp from a fresh-cut leaf helps the work of healing cuts and burns. It is used in shampoo, sunburn lotions, and a burn ointment that has been used by the government after testing at Los Alamos proving ground under the auspices of the U.S. Atomic Energy Commission.

The First Aid Miracle Plant

If you have never heard of the first aid plant, ask a few of your neighbors. You should soon find someone who can tell you their experiences. They may call it the "Burn Plant," but the official name is Aloe Vera.

The Wonders of Nature

Aloe Vera is just one of nature's wonders in her botanical kingdom, with about one and a half million species. It is a mysterious world still waiting for its countless secrets to be discovered. For decades, scientists have been prowling over mountainsides, cutting their way through jungles, scanning deserts, coastlines and wastelands all over the world, keeping their eyes on flowers, herbs, plants, and trees. They have been eagerly making notes and listening carefully to legends, miraculous stories, and even to strange superstitions of natives. Scientists are continuing to burrow deeply into ancient writings and folklore to rediscover forgotten plants and herbs that may possess remarkable medical properties.

It is no wonder that today one-fourth of the two billion prescriptions filled in the United States contain botanical derivatives such as alkaloids, glycosides, steroids, etc. It is estimated the total value of drugs derived from higher plants exceeds three billion dollars a year. There is hardly a food, beverage, or cosmetic preparation which does not contain spices, essential oils, enzymes, vitamins, plant hydrolloids, or other botanical ingredients.

Aloe Vera, in contrast to many other long forgotten medicinal plants, has retained a respected place in the professional medicine cabinet down through the ages. Unfortunately, however, an understanding of only a few of its many uses were remembered; the rest were often neglected and finally forgotten. That has been unfortunate, for it is becoming increasingly evident that much unnecessary suffering, scarring, incapacity, and expense of many patients has been the result.

ALOE VERA—WHAT IS IT?

Aloe Vera (usually pronounced a´low veer´a) is also known by many grateful laymen as the "Medicine Plant," "Burn Plant," "First Aid Plant" or "Miracle Plant." Its botanical name is *Aloe Barbadenisis*. In Spanish its name is Sa'vila. In Sanscrit, it is Ghrita-kumari. It is Jadam in Malaysia, Lu-hui in Chinese, Erva Babosa in Portuguese, but in Greek, Latin, Italian, German, Russian, French and Hawaiian, it is Aloe, with the "e" being pronounced as a long "a." "Vera" is a Latin word meaning "true" and was so named in ancient times because it was thought that this particular species of Aloe had the best medicinal properties. However, in recent years a few of the other Aloe species have been found to work equally as well.

Actually, the Aloe family contains over two hundred different species which grow in the dry regions of' Africa, Asia, Europe, and the Americas. Aloe resembles cactus in appearance but is actually a perennial succulent belonging to the Lily (Liliaceae) family. These plants are characterized by stiff, lance-shaped leaves with a sharp apex and spiny edges. The colors of these leaves vary from grey to bright green and some species even have striped leaves. They bloom in early spring as a dense cluster of yellow or red tube-shaped flowers produced on the very top of a leafless stem. The Aloe family is not a large one and belongs to a larger class of plants known as the "Xeroids," so called because they possess the ability to close their stomata completely to avoid loss of water. They can survive long periods of drought stress. Almost all xeroids have a special chemical makeup which closes any wound almost immediately so the plant will not lose its precious water. The wound then heals with almost miraculous rapidity and the plant begins to grow in another direction. Ancient man may have observed this and reasoned that if it worked for the plant it would work for him.

The History of Aloe Vera

For centuries Aloe Vera and its medicinal cousins have been used extensively in many cultures because of their apparently magical effectiveness for treating burns, healing wounds, and relieving aches and pains, including the "heartbreak of psoriasis" where, when used regularly, it reduces scaling and itching, greatly improving appearance. Historical documents of the Egyptians, Romans, Greeks, Algerians, Moroccans, Tunisians, Arabians, Indians, and Chinese report of its medicinal and cosmetic uses. According to numerous traditions, Cleopatra attributed her irresistible charm and beauty to the use of Aloe gel.

The earliest recording is 1500 B.C. in the *Papyrus Ebers*, the original copies of which are safeguarded in Leipzig University. These Egyptian papers state that the many medicinal values of Aloe were widely acclaimed and had been for many centuries before. The author of the famed *Greek Herbal*, Dioscorides, of the first century A.D., made a lengthy, detailed report of its many applications for wounds, binding, insomnia, stomach disorders, pain, constipation, hemorrhoids, itching, headache, loss of hair, mouth and gum diseases, kidney ailments, blistering, skin care, sunburn, blemishes, etc.

Historians state that Aristotle persuaded Alexander the Great to conquer the island of Socroto off the east coast of Africa for the purpose of obtaining sufficient amounts of Aloe as a wound healing agent for his soldiers. Other ancient records describe its application for skin care, protection against the sun, wind, fire and cold, healing of small wounds, relieving insect stings and bites, scratches, scalds, bruises, cuts, abrasions, urticaria, acne, poison ivy, blemishes, allergic conditions, welts, fistula, irritations due to faulty diet, ulcerated skin lesions, eczema, and otherwise damaged skin.

It is mentioned in John 19:39 as part of the mixture being used for the anointing of the body of Jesus after his death.

Recent History of Aloe Vera

Except for the powdered Aloe sap used as a cathartic, Aloe Vera juice fell into disuse in the West as the seat of civilization moved to the temperate zones where the tropical plant could not survive the freezing winters. Other remedies were substituted and since most modern medicine comes from the culture of the temperate zone, it has been only recently that Aloe Vera has been "rediscovered" and has started to come back into more common use. Ironically enough, it was the invention of the X-ray and the atom bomb which again focused scientific attention upon the plant. Radiation burns caused skin ulcerations which were nearly incurable until doctors began trying the old folk remedy of the Aloe Vera leaf. It usually worked better than anything else. However, since no one knew how to preserve the juice so that it would not spoil, the leaves of the plant had to be shipped in from the tropics.

Rodney M. Stockton, a chemical engineer vacationing in Florida in 1942, suffered a severe sunburn. He was amazed when some friends spread the fresh Aloe Vera juice on his skin, giving instant relief and bringing prompt healing. In 1947, Mr. Stockton moved to Florida to work seriously on the problem of stabilizing the healing gel. He was successful and began manufacturing products. A report in *Industrial Medicine and Surgery Journal*, August 1959, showed that the AloCreme ointment he developed could change a deep thermal burn within 48 hours to a minor second-degree burn by the rapid regeneration of tissues. The burns, being control-tested on rabbits, healed 30 percent faster than when using regular ointments. Most important, healing took place without gross scar tissue.

During the last thirty years, research programs on Aloe Vera have been undertaken in many parts of the world. Surprisingly, the Soviet Union has been the leader by far. Even in the West, many intensive studies have been carried out to determine what made it so effective. As its fame began to spread, numerous companies were formed to produce Aloe Vera products. There was great expectation in the late fifties and early sixties that soon everyone in the country would be taking advantage of this amazing gift of nature.

However, such was not the case. Growth in its popularity has been continuous but relatively slow. Then in the last several years, a groundswell of awareness has taken place. Each year more millions of Americans are getting to appreciate, at least to some degree, what Aloe Vera can do. It is a remarkable plant to be excited about, for people enjoy sharing good news. For example, the late Will Geer, the grandfather on the Walton TV show, when being a guest on the *Johnny Carson Show*, would often bring an Aloe Vera plant and joyfully praise its values. Other national TV Shows, such as *Dinah Shore*, have had special guests relate personal experiences. More and more articles in newspapers and magazines are appearing. As Aloe Vera rises in fame, many cosmetic firms are starting to add Aloe Vera to their product line, such as moisturizers, cleansers, face-lifts, and even deodorant as well as shaving and shampoo preparations.

ALOE VERA—HOW AND WHY IT HEALS

Due to this growth in commercial applications, a report was included in the *Drugs and Cosmetics Journal*, June 1977, produced by a noted consultant, Dr. Albert T. Leun, Ph.D. He states the following:

"During the past three years, there has been considerably revived interest in Aloe Vera as a cosmetic ingredient. Several major cosmetic and consumer product companies have incorporated it into their products and others currently are at the developmental or pilot stage with their own lines of Aloe Vera cosmetics... All take advantage of the age-old reputation of Aloe Vera as a skin-healer, skin softener and moisturizer... It is commonly believed that the moisturizing emollient and healing properties of Aloe gel are due to the polysaccharides present. The major polysaccharide present has been determined to be a glucomannan. Other polysaccharides containing galactose and uronic acids as well as pentoses are also present. It is probable that the gel's beneficial properties are not due to the polysaccharides alone, but rather from a synergistic effect of these compounds with other substances present in the gel."

If that sounds a little complex, it is no wonder. After three decades of intensive analysis, the laboratories are only partially able to explain Aloe Vera's incredible non-toxic potency. The gel is a most ingenious mixture of antibiotic, astringent, and coagulating agents, while also being a pain and scar inhibitor and a growth stimulator. The scientific term for this last characteristic is biogenic stimulator. One famous German research pharmacist, Freytag, calls it a "wound hormone." In simple terms, it accelerates the healing of injured surfaces. Russian scientists first began to experiment with the "wound hormone" on rats and rabbits. They reported that artificially induced skin lesions on these animals responded rapidly. The same was even true on plant wounds. It was shortly thereafter that they discovered its effectiveness on the treatment of human ulcers, including peptic, dendrite karatitis and cutaneous leishmaniasias.

The intensive and broadly based research done in Russia has not been matched in any of the Western democracies. However, we have still been moving ahead, as can be seen by references to positive applications reported in such authoritative medical publications as the *Journal of Pharmaceutical Science, Oral Surgery, Cancer, Industrial Medicine and Surgery*, and the *International Journal of Dermatology*. We have listed many of these articles in the appendix. Also available is a book published by the Aloe Vera Research Institute covering excerpts from many of these reports. These scientific articles often describe the ailments in technical, medical terms, such as alopecia areata, kraurois vulvae, periodontosis, achorrhea, and aplmar eczema. But the reports also deal with familiar old names we can quickly recognize such as acne, anemia, burns, constipation, heartburn, leg ulcer, peptic ulcers, poison ivy, psoriasis, scalds, sunburn and tuberculosis.

I have seen the bulging files of testimonials accumulated by several manufacturers of Aloe Vera products giving grateful acknowledgements of the personal benefits people report they have experienced. For many external applications, these reports indicate results that are often rapid and amazing. For internal use, the results are usually slower but, according to the many letters, no less dramatic. There are those who feel that a normal, healthy person drinking Aloe Vera gel is more likely to stay healthy than a non-user. Whatever your own conclusions may be regarding the curative powers of this plant, there is no doubt that you will find it truly unique in its appearance, history, and many possible uses.

A Point of Caution

The Food and Drug Administration (FDA) has not specifically approved Aloe Vera for any ailment other than minor first aid. However, we know of no restrictions on Aloe Vera or the way it can be used, other than the making of claims. It is being sold throughout the country for both internal and external use in great quantities (over 100,000 gallons a month). While many thousands of people are grateful users, until the required documentation and clinical research has been completed, we do not say that Aloe Vera will cure anything.

Aloe Vera is widely recognized for being harmless, for having no bad side effects. However, if a person stopped using one medication which was helping and substituted a treatment which was not helpful, then it could be to the person's disadvantage. Therefore, we strongly urge all who have a medical problem to obtain qualified professional attention.

Possible Allergy to Aloe Vera

There is nothing that some people are not allergic to. A few people, probably less than one out of a hundred, are allergic to Aloe Vera. Such people will report the opposite results. Allergy is usually indicated by a stinging sensation or a mild rash. This will usually show up within a few minutes, so anyone can do a quick test. Put a little juice, either from the plant or a bottle, on the under arm or behind the ear. If stinging or a rash occurs within a few minutes, do not use Aloe Vera.

Fortunately, many people who have a host of allergic reactions from other things find that the application of Aloe Vera reduces or eliminates the effect of the other reactions. So for most people, Aloe Vera is an anti-allergenic.

11

Burns and Scalds

Burns are described in four categories:

First Degree – skin not broken,
Second Degree – blisters and skin broken,
Third Degree – all layers of skin destroyed and open wound,
Fourth Degree – skin charred.

All burns can be serious and should not be treated lightly, but particularly those beyond first degree. Besides the pain and possible scarring, there can be great danger of infection. Medical attention is important.

Aloe Vera is excellent for first aid treatment. It can stop pain and reduce the chance of infection and scarring while greatly enhancing the healing process. In addition, since Aloe Vera is quickly absorbed, it is not in the way of any later medical treatment that may be required.

Aloe Vera ointments are particularly designed for continuous treatment of burns since they contain lubricants to help offset the astringent aspects of the juice.

For thousands of years people have used the soothing juice from Aloe Vera for relief from even the most serious burns by keeping the wound continually wet with the juice. After continuous application, when the pulp would seem to become dry, they would merely scratch the surface of the pulp to release more juice until the pulp was all gone. By keeping the wound wet for the first 48 hours, marvelous recoveries have been reported, with little or no pain or scarring. However, it should be remembered that each of us is different and each burn is different. For example, if the burn is caused or associated with acid, it is vital that the wound be thoroughly washed before treatment.

Sunburn

Prevention of sunburn is easy with use of an Aloe Vera lotion containing a sun screen. Apply before exposure and after swimming or extensive sweating. A good Aloe Vera suntan lotion blocks out over 90 percent of the burning rays but allows over 75 percent of the tanning rays to reach the skin.

For treatment of mild to fair sunburn, cover frequently with Aloe Vera juice, either from a pump spray bottle, by cotton pad, or directly from the leaf. Repeat often. This reduces pain, stiffness, and the amount of peeling. Aloe Vera ointment may be preferred over the straight juice by some.

For the treatment of a heavy sunburn, time is critical. Giving first aid as soon as possible reduces complications because burned cells heat up and burn more skin cells. Keep the skin wet with juice. Aloe Vera is an astringent and will tend to dry the skin unless kept wet or used along with some skin oil, such as olive oil or baby oil. Bandaging the open leaf on critical areas can be helpful. Using Aloe Vera ointment, since it contains oils, is also encouraged. Remember, before using Aloe Vera for the first time on a person, give the allergy test. Heavy sunburn can be very serious and professional medical attention is recommended.

Cuts and Wounds

Aloe Vera was famous even before the days of Alexander the Great for aiding the body to heal wounds. Users have claimed that it inhibits infection, enhances healing, and reduces scarring. The old home remedy still used in much of the world is to clean the wound, put Aloe Vera pulp in the wound, close it up tightly, and keep the bandage soaked in Aloe Vera juice—or if available, Aloe Vera ointment. Many people attest to the ease of removing bandages, rapid healing, and little or no scarring.

Digestive Problems

When a person has a medical problem, he should consult a physician. Pain in the abdomen may be serious and can be caused by a great variety of very different things.

In many areas of the world where medical attention is not available, Aloe Vera is one of the first things people try. They claim that it is often the answer, but obviously, not always. Many people in the States take it if they have constipation, and also for dysentery. Not being a medicine, it seems to help the digestive organs perk up and do the job they are designed to do. There have been many reports that it is effective in cases of colitis and other inflammations of the digestive track. There are also reports by people who felt it helped them with kidney infection.

Taking a tablespoon or two of the juice or gel several times a day does seem to act like a general tonic and mild regulator of the bowels. The Aloe Vera juice from the pulp is not a real laxative but the sap is. The sap—the yellow bitter fluid which flows between the skin and the pulp—is a cathartic. That is why some people place the green peelings of the leaf in a jar of water in the refrigerator and drink a little once or twice a week as a natural remedy. The strength is determined by the amount of peel in the jar. They fill the jar each time the physic is used.

Hair and Scalp Care

Soaps tend to leave film on the hair and scalp while detergent concentrates do not. Aloe Vera has been added to good detergent concentrate shampoos to give healing qualities to the scalp while the cleansers do their work.

Hair and scalp conditions vary so much in different people that each person must find out what works best for themselves. Some Aloe Vera shampoos have built-in hair conditioners to make the hair more manageable and fuller in texture. Other shampoos require a separate hair conditioner. There are advantages to each, so people should discover their own preference.

Before all these wonder products, straight Aloe Vera juice was used for the hair as a shampoo, hair set, and conditioner, with remarkable results for both the hair and the scalp. It is said that the Indians in Mexico wet their hair at night with the juice right from the plant, allowed it to dry, and then in the morning, rinsed with water, which even suds somewhat. This process reportedly added luster, richness, and manageability to the hair. As reported in the July 1978 issue of *Let's Live*, Esperanza Aguilar has used straight Aloe Vera from the plant as a wave set in her beauty shop since the 1930s. She explains: "The gel dries quickly, improves hair sheen, and helps scalp abrasions." She calls it her *fortuna bien*.

Diseases of the scalp are often treated directly by Aloe Vera juice. A recent medical report in the *International Journal of Dermatology* gave very positive results.

Hemorrhoids and Bleeding Piles

Aloe Vera has been respected for thousands of years for its ability to bring relief from hemorrhoidal itching and pain. A chunk of peeled pulp the size of half a finger was inserted into the rectum. That still works but is a little hard to do unless the chunk is frozen stiff to provide rigidity. Now that Aloe Vera ointments are available, they are much handier. The application is easiest to apply by putting ointment on the index finger and inserting it gently into the rectum to work the ointment well into the area. Some people put a few tablespoons of Aloe Vera juice in a syringe, depositing the liquid in the rectum. A combination of both juice and ointment has been useful in different cases.

Applications have been repeated as often as desired, but at least after each bowel movement, after a bath, and before retiring. Relief was usually immediate but if not, using the pulp of the plant as a suppository was the most powerful way. People often keep up the treatment for a while even after the symptoms are gone.

Infections

Medical reports stress the absence of infection when treating wounds with Aloe Vera. As a home remedy, a split leaf was bound over an infected wound to work like a poultice and showed remarkable improvement within twelve hours. Many people report the same results from Aloe Vera ointment when very generously applied.

Poison Ivy, Poison Oak, and Allergies

Since Aloe Vera is a pain inhibitor, it greatly reduces the problem of itching. It also enhances the healing of rashes and sores. Thus it is a very effective treatment for the agony of poison ivy and poison oak. It is also helpful for many other types of allergies, so it is well worth a try for anyone suffering from skin problems. One would frequently spray the juice on the area or apply ointment, whichever works best.

Psoriasis and Eczematous Rashes

It is said that psoriasis cannot be cured but it can be controlled. Often these situations are both an internal as well as an external abnormality and medical attention is recommended. Those who state that Aloe Vera was effective for them have often taken Aloe Vera internally (one to two tablespoons once or twice a day) as well as applying the juice to the affected area. The juice was applied at least twice a day and continued even after most of the inflammation was gone. The Aloe Vera ointments may be better, unless a person is allergic to one of the added ingredients in the ointment. Remember, Aloe Vera juice is an astringent and may cause the skin to dry, thus treatment might be accompanied with baby oil or other lubricants.

Scar Removal

Many people attest to the effectiveness of Aloe Vera in the reduction and possible removal of minor scars. They applied Aloe Vera juice morning and night. One should not be impatient because the effect is not fast. Usually several months, even up to six, is necessary. Some have reported that vitamin E was also effective and have combined the two applications.

Stretch Marks from Pregnancy

Many women during pregnancy have applied Aloe Vera to the skin around the abdomen to aid the skin in adapting to the unusual stresses during pregnancy. Then following delivery, they have continued application to enhance the return to normalcy. Their reports are very positive and they encourage other mothers to do the same.

Varicose Veins

Varicose veins can be very painful and serious and should receive proper medical attention. Since Aloe Vera is considered by scientists to be a biogenic stimulator and a "wound hormone," many people have tried the external application of Aloe Vera juice to the afflicted area. In some cases, at least, the results were very positive. Certainly, all should agree, it will do no harm.

Skin Cancer

Skin cancer is a serious medical problem, of course, and should have medical attention. There are many reports of total elimination by applying Aloe Vera juice 2 to 4 times a day for several months.

Scrapes and Abrasions

Since scrapes are often quite painful, even the application of Aloe Vera ointment may be too painful. In such a case, either spray the juice on with a pump applicator or tenderly apply a split leaf, sliding it gently over the area. Reapplication should be done frequently during the first 24 hours. When the sensitivity of the wound has decreased, the person may want to start using the Aloe Vera ointment. People are greatly impressed with the rather painless and very rapid recovery of these usually painful injuries.

Stings by Insects, Jellyfish, Stinging Nettle, etc.

When bitten by a bee, ant, wasp, yellow jacket, scorpion, centipede, or other insects, time is very important. If you have the plant, split a leaf immediately and lay the leaf over the area. Many people report a gradual reduction in pain, little or no swelling, and quick recovery. People have different degrees of sensitivity to stings, however, so medical attention may be indicated.

If the plant is not available, then use the bottled juice or ointment. If first aid is not applied fairly quickly, the possible benefits are greatly reduced. Since the most frequent and least painful of all bites is the mosquito, a pump-spray container of juice is a very handy thing to have when out of doors on summer evenings.

Ulcers

Ulcers are very serious and should be given medical attention. Clinical research using Aloe Vera reported in the medical journals has been very encouraging. Since Aloe Vera appears to have no negative side effects, it has been tried by many people. Most of these people say they took the juice or the gel four times a day, preferably half an hour before each meal and upon going to bed. To ease the taste, it is often taken with milk. The amount would vary by the individual, but most took from 2 to 4 tablespoons each time, at first, until the symptoms had diminished, then reduced the amount by half. They found it wise to stay on their bland diet for a period of several months and then gradually tested their way back to a normal diet.

When some people have found that the commercial juice or gel was not handling their case, they have started eating chunks of the pulp directly from the leaf. This was done by taking a thick leaf, peeling off the skin, and rinsing the yellow sap from the pulp, then swallowing the chunks of pulp. Some liquefy the chunks in a blender and drink it. If the taste is bitter, it is only because all the yellow sap which flows between the green skin and the pulp was not removed.

Arthritis

Many thousands of people who have been drinking a little Aloe Vera each day report that they suffer much less from their arthritis. To what extent this occurs and on which types of arthritis, present research is attempting to discover. Whether it will be useful to you can only be known by your own experience.

Most people who report some relief from arthritic symptoms say they drink one or two tablespoons at a time, two to four times a day. Most prefer drinking the Aloe Vera gel while others prefer the juice, but all say either is easier to take when refrigerated. Usually it is taken with a little fruit or vegetable juice, followed by a drink of juice or water.

While some people report encouraging results right away, many find that a real difference does not take place until the second month. So a minimum two-month test is encouraged for those really interested in checking Aloe Vera out. At a rate of 4 tablespoons a day, a gallon will last one person two months. Once the painful symptoms diminish to the extent that they are no longer a serious problem, one tablespoon morning and evening is often used as a maintenance program.

For those who feel that they cannot afford the bottled juice or gel, the old-fashioned way can be used to make a drink directly from the plant. It is done by dicing up a leaf from the Aloe Vera plant, placing the pieces in a refrigerated jar of water, and adding more water as it is consumed. The bitter taste soon leaves. However, since the bitterness comes from the sap and not the juice, this can be eliminated by peeling the skin from off the colorless pulp, rinsing the pulp of all sap residue, and placing it in the jar of water.

For aching joints and muscles, Aloe Vera is also very effective for temporary relief by rubbing it on the outer surface of the skin. Relief is often felt within a few minutes and can be repeated frequently with no bad side effects. Aloe Vera massage creme is the subject of many favorable reports.

Brown Skin Spots

Brown skin spots come as we grow older and appear on those areas of skin which have been exposed to the sun. Many people have described the process by which Aloe Vera reduced or removed the spot after several months of twice-daily applications of Aloe Vera juice or gel. From these reports we gather that the results are not fast but they are definite.

Acne

Acne is caused by deep infection in oil-clogged pores. This occurs frequently in adolescence because the skin is going through a changing process. The steps necessary to prevent long-term damage are as follows:

Good Cleansing: Morning and night the skin should be scrubbed well. When ordinary soaps are too harsh or cause reactions, Aloe Vera soap has often been found useful. Ordinary cleansing creams should not be used because they contain oil. An excess of oil is often one of the problems.

Apply Aloe Vera: Aloe Vera does a remarkable job of counteracting infection, stimulating the tissues and healing without scarring. The juice can be applied by using either the leaf of the plant directly, the bottled gel, or Aloe Vera ointment. Remember, if you are using an Aloe Vera ointment, a little goes a long way.

Treating Sores: Pimples and other sores can be treated with Aloe Vera ointment or the salve, Kleer. These products can enhance healing and reduce the possibility of scars.

Removal of Old Acne Scars: Aloe Vera is effective in gradually reducing old scars if used regularly and with patience. Putting on a little Aloe Vera juice morning and night for as long as necessary, even six months, is a small price to pay for a greatly improved complexion. Not only will it help to reduce scars, but it will also give greater health and color to the skin. However, since Aloe Vera is a natural astringent, it will tend to be drying. For oily skin, this can be desired but for dry skin, Aloe Vera needs to be accompanied by one of the fine Aloe Vera moisturizing cremes.

Animal First Aid

There are many ways that Aloe Vera can be used for treating the ailments of our family pets. For example, people say they have added Aloe Vera to dog food for remarkable improvement in crippling arthritis. Digestive problems have also received favorable results after a number of other approaches had failed. Treating hot spots on long-haired dogs worked overnight when everything else had failed. The deformity called "Collie Nose," where a dog is born without the black leather-type skin on the top of its nose, has been helped by treating it with Aloe Vera Suntan Lotion to prevent sunburn and blistering, and promote healing. Handling wounds and infections are probably the most common. So again, the nice thing about Aloe Vera is that it works in so many ways, but even when it doesn't, it does no harm.

Aloe Vera Health Drink

Many people who are in excellent health make a habit of drinking a tablespoon of Aloe Vera juice or gel every morning, along with a little fruit juice. The reason many people give is that they seem to have more energy, their digestion is better, and they believe they will stay healthier. They state that if Aloe Vera will help the body take care of ulcers, constipation, colitis, and possibly even arthritis, then it certainly might be helpful in preventing these and similar conditions. Traditionally, Aloe Vera has also been acclaimed for being effective in the very early stages of digestive cancer. If this is so, and it is certainly possible that it is, then a little Aloe Vera every day would be one of the wisest things we could be doing—especially since it wouldn't be doing any harm.

Incidentally, the Russians tested Aloe Vera to see if it increased the body's ability to handle harmful substances.

Tests were conducted on rabbits. After being given Aloe Vera for 30 days, a third of the rabbits were able to survive normally deadly doses of strychnine whereas no rabbits without Aloe Vera had been able to survive. This is another indication that the natural protective functions of the body are stimulated by this wonderful plant.

Sinus

Sinus has to do with pressures in the sinus cavities which extend throughout most of the face. There are inhalers and other medications that reduce the discomfort of sinus, but they must not be used too often. Although Aloe Vera is not as dramatic as such things as antihistamines, it has been used by many people with considerable benefit. Most people take an empty inhaler, remove the nipple with a pair of pliers, clean the bottle thoroughly, then fill it about ⅔ full with stabilized Aloe Vera juice. After the nipple with its little tube has been refitted, one has a nice inexpensive inhaler. People who have tried it report that they find it more effective to use it regularly, even before the sinus starts bothering them. Since it is not a powerful decongestant, it is less helpful when the condition becomes acute.

Asthma

One of the old remedies for asthma was to boil some Aloe Vera leaves in a pan of water and breathe in the vapor. The results earned Aloe Vera a revered place as a home remedy for asthma. The modern application would be to put some stabilized Aloe Vera juice in an atomizer. This also has the advantage of allowing the breathing of cold mist since some asthmatics cannot handle steam mist very well.

Sore Throat

Many people find Aloe Vera useful for reducing the pain of a sore throat. Since Aloe Vera is not a medicine, it is one gargle that can be swallowed. As one is gargling, little sips can be swallowed in order to get deeper penetration down the throat. Because Aloe Vera is not a strong antiseptic, it will be less dramatic than some medications, but since it can be done frequently, the overall effect has been reported to be excellent.

Eye and Ear Drops

Of course, the eyes and ears are two of the most delicate organs of the body and should be given proper medical attention when disorders occur. As a home remedy, Aloe Vera has been used for centuries. A few drops in an aching ear have often brought relief immediately, or sometimes increased the pain a little for a while before bringing relief. Many have acclaimed it as a fine eye drop solution. Some have mixed Aloe Vera juice half and half with water to reduce its acidity so it won't smart as much.

Taking Care of Your Aloe Vera Plant

Size of Plant. It is often said incorrectly that a plant has to be three to four years old before it is potent enough to be used for healing. Actually, even a very young plant has considerable potency. However, the strength does increase with age and one should have at least one mature plant around the home. For this reason we encourage people to purchase as large an Aloe Vera as they have room for in the home. The plants usually grow very slowly in the house.

Indoors and Outdoors. Aloe Vera turns brown in harsh sunlight so it should be kept in indirect light. It will freeze so it must be protected when danger of heavy frost exists. Other than that, it grows faster outside than inside, but most people grow Aloe Vera as an indoor ornamental plant.

Watering. Aloe Vera is a succulent. This means that it is in greater danger of overwatering than underwatering. It should be allowed to become fairly dry before watering. During the winter months, watering should be light, such as only a cup or two, since drying out will be slow. In the summer, the pot can be really soaked. Be sure there is a drainage hole in the pot since the roots will rot off when exposed to long periods of wet soil.

Repotting. Aloe Vera can stand being root-bound, so repotting is not necessary until the upper plant gets top-heavy. When a plant gets root-bound, it will send out more new shoots or pups. If these are not taken out for replanting when they are 3 to 4 inches high, they will suck the life from the mother plant, which will get bright green and spread its leaves horizontally rather than vertically. The plants will grow in any kind of soil but good drainage is essential. The pups should be repotted when large enough, watered well, and not watered again for about 3 weeks, forcing new roots to seek water. The transplanted pup may turn grey or brown for a while, which is normal. New pups make wonderful presents.

Cutting Off Part of a Leaf. It does not harm the plant to harvest part or all of a leaf since the wound is quickly sealed and healed. However, since the leaf will not grow back, one should cut on the leaves closest to the ground. These are also the oldest, therefore the most potent medicinally.

Symptoms of Poor Plant Care

1. Leaves lie flat instead of upright: Usually caused by insufficient light. Although Aloe Vera turns brown in harsh sunlight, it does need a fair amount of light.

2. Leaves are thin and curled: Not being watered well enough, thus using up its own liquid.

3. Leaves brown: Too much direct sunshine.

4. Very slow growth: Probable causes might be too alkaline water or soil, too damp for too long, not enough light, or too much fertilizer.

5. Disease or infestation: This is almost non-existent here in the temperate zone.

USING AN ALOE VERA LEAF
FOR EXTERNAL USE

What Leaf to Use? Always use the lowest leaves, the ones closest to the ground, first. The bottom leaves are older and larger, thus have more juice and greater potency. Also, since the plant grows from the center and the cut leaves do not grow back, the plant will still retain its beauty and continued growth.

How to Cut a Leaf: After cutting off the portion of the leaf you want with a sharp knife, trim the thorny edges from the severed portion, then slice the leaf across its width, like filleting a fish. The inner, exposed surfaces will reveal the transparent, gooey gel which is ready to be applied directly to the afflicted area. Use it generously. It will be absorbed by the skin within several minutes.

How Long Will a Leaf Last? If the gel is being applied over a large area, like a sunburn, it may soon seem to be exhausted of gel by running dry. This is only a surface appearance because the remaining gel is held captive in small elongated cells underneath which are still intact. After the gel from the first layer of ruptured cells has run dry, scratch the surface with a clean knife to rupture more cells, releasing more juice. This can be continued until there is nothing but green skin left. A partially used leaf can be wrapped in foil or plastic wrap and refrigerated, where it will last for days.

Is the Leaf Better Than Aloe Vera Products? The juice direct from the leaf is usually more potent than the processed and stabilized juice or gel obtainable in bottled form, but the bottled product is usually potent enough to do the job and is much more convenient. Also, the plant when used alone has some limitations. Since Aloe Vera, by itself, is an astringent, it tends to be drying to the skin. Chemists have found it advantageous to combine it with other active ingredients, such as vitamins A and E, lanolin and other healing elements, to broaden and intensify its effectiveness. Thus, we ordinarily recommend the enriched Aloe Vera products according to their specific applications. So if one is using the plant and it is not quite doing the job, an appropriate product might be tried. In contrast, if one is not getting full effectiveness from a product, we recommend that before giving up on Aloe Vera, the plant might be tried.

USING THE ALOE VERA PLANT
FOR INTERNAL USE

Is It Better to Use the Fresh Plant or Bottled Juice? If one has decided to try Aloe Vera for internal benefit, the commercial, stabilized juice or gel is the most convenient way to do so. It is relatively inexpensive since only small amounts are taken at a time. It is also convenient, and if kept cold, nearly tasteless. However, since the direct plant is somewhat more potent than the bottled juice, some have found it necessary to go directly to the plant before getting the results they wanted in very difficult cases.

How to Consume the Plant Directly: If one has ever tried to eat an Aloe Vera leaf, the experience is usually very difficult. The reason is that although the colorless pulp is nearly tasteless, the yellow sap which flows between the pulp and the skin is very bitter. So to prepare the pulp for internal consumption, peel the green skin off from the pulp. Since some pulp is peeled off with the rind, most of the sap is also removed. Rinse the pulp off with cool water to remove any remaining sap. The remaining chunks of pulp, which resemble colorless jellyfish, can be eaten directly or turned into liquid in a blender. It is not bitter but has a slight taste which is unique, and some compare it to parsley or a medicine flavor. The taste leaves quickly if followed by a drink of water or other liquids.

Medical References on Effective Use of Aloe Vera

Current status of Aloe Vera research by Dr. G. Gjerstad, Director, Alkaloid Biosynthesis Research, University of Texas, in the *American Journal of Pharmacy*, p. 58-64, Vol. 140.

Used on burns and scalds by J. L. Crew, M.D. in *Minnesota Medicine*, Vol. 20, p. 670-3 and Vol. 22, p. 538-9. Also research report by B. Rovath, M.D. in *Ind. Medicine & Surgery*, p. 364-8, Vol. 28.

For peptic ulcer therapy by Julian J. Blitz, O.D. et. al., in *Journal of American Osteopathic Assoc.*, Vol. 62, p. 73 1 -5. Also book by J. G. Allen, M.D., University of Chicago Press.

Research on antibacteriostatic effects by L. J. Lorenzetti, et al., College of Pharmacy, Ohio State University in *Journal of Pharm. Science*, p. 1287, Vol. 53.

Used on leg ulcers, acne vulgaris, seborrhea and alopacia by E. E. Zawahry, M.D., Professor of Dermatology, Faculty of Medicine, Cairo University, et al., *International Journal of Dermatology*, Jan/Feb 1973, p. 68-73.

For postoperative treatment in dental surgery by E. G. Bovik, D.D.S. in Texas *Dental Journal*, p. 13, Vol. 84.

For inflammatory lesions in the mouth by E. R. Zimmermann, D.D.S., et al., College of Dentistry, Baylor University, in Oral Surgery, p. 122-7, Jan. 1969.

For radiation caused ulcers in mouth by F. B. Mandeville, M.D., Professor of Radiology, Medical College of Virginia, in *Radiation*, p. 598-9, Vol. 32.

For radiation caused skin ulcers by C. E. Collins, M.D. in *Journal of Roentgenology*, p. 396-7, Vol. 33: 1. Also by C. S. Wright, M.D., in *Journal of American Medical Association*, p. 1363-4, Vol. 106. Also by A. B. Loveman, M.D., in *Archives of Dermatology & Syph.*, p. 838-43, Vol. 36.

Used in oriental dermatology by H. N. Cole, M.D. and K. D. Chen, M.D., in *Archives of Dermatology and Syph.*, p. 250, Vol. 47.

Index

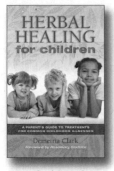
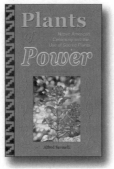
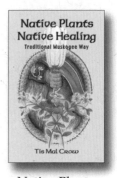
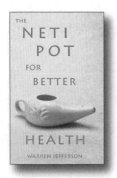
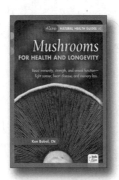
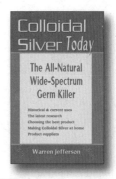